YOUR GUIDE
to positive life

WORKBOOK III
Brain gymnastics for adult

KATARZYNA DOROSZ

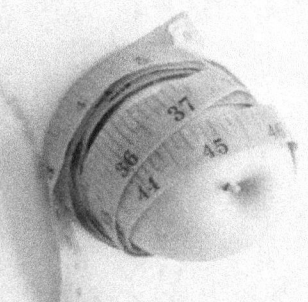

Here's an educational workbook for you:

„Your Guide to Positive Life.
Volume III: Brain gymnastics for adults"

This is your next booklet in the series of original exercises which will help you discover the power that flows from the inside.

As we work through it, you will:
- learn to activate your natural improvement mechanisms,
- increase your physical and intellectual activity,
- master your relaxation skills,
- learn to handle stress,
- improve short- and long-term memory,
- develop abstract thinking and the ability to clearly express your thoughts,
- learn to influence the quality of your relationships through, amongst other skills, learning to communicate properly, developing your understanding of social situations and problem solving skills.

What if I told you that simple gymnastics of your brain can help you become more open to the world and the people around you? How would you feel about that?

This is your time. Take control of your
life – health – relationships – dreams

Remember: you are doing it for yourself!

I wish you good luck in discovering yourself!
Kasia Dorosz

Table of contents

Introduction..1
Support your brain...2
Two hemispheres, one human being...3
Exercise and remember..5
New activities as a remedy for better memory...........................6
Activating exercises...9
Stretching exercises...15
Creative exercises...23

Copyright © Katarzyna Dorosz

Introduction

If you have worked through my previous guides, you need to know that this one is very different.

The volume you are holding is divided into two main parts:

I. Theoretical, on the brain and its functioning.

First of all, I want to show you what a treasure it is that you carry inside you every day. With a little bit of systematic work and commitment you can really achieve a lot. In this part, in addition to essential knowledge, you'll also find incentive to work on your memory and shape new skills.

II. Practical, a collection of exercises.

All the physical exercises presented here are based on the work of dr Paul Dennison, an American educator who has developed a method of supporting our brains through movement. I have added several other creative and linguistic exercises which can positively enhance your brain function, and thus your whole life.

Let this guide become actual gymnastics for your brain. However, remember what we have already worked on through the previous volumes. **Practice daily gratitude, meditation and physical activity.** Scrupulously record all changes in your life in your diary. Remember to write down the answers to the following questions:
- What am I grateful for today?
- What good did I do today?
- What have I learned today?
- How much did I exercise today? What did I eat?

Review your notes regularly to celebrate the achievement of your goals.

SUPPORT YOUR BRAIN

You've probably heard that with age, the ability to acquire new skills decreases and the brain is not as agile as before? I have good news for you – none of this is true! We already have evidence that the brain, regardless of age, **creates millions of new connections between neurons in every second of your life**. This is a huge potential that you can use to learn!

Once you know this, **there is only one thing left to do – find motivation to acquire new skills.**

> **Did you know ...?**
> The brain weighs approx 1-2.5 kg
> and has about 1,5 l of capacity. Although it only
> constitutes 2% of the human body,
> it uses up as much as 20% of its energy.

In order to help your brain, remember to:
- Constantly take advantage of new cognitive opportunities.
  Gain new skills, perform various physical exercises, challenge yourself!

- Get the right amount of sleep.
  Despite its constant work, your brain can rest and analyze all the information it received during the day when you sleep.

- Exercise.
  It's the best way to oxygenate your brain.

- Have an active social life.
  We are made to build relationships, which are the fuel that provides us with energy to live.

- Keep a balanced diet.
  Make sure that your meals are rich in carbohydrates, fats, proteins, iron and vitamins (mainly B, A, C, E), as well as omega-3 fatty acids. Avoid processed foods.

These basic things, which I constantly encourage you to bear in mind, will improve your memory and concentration, which in turn will improve your mood and increase your self-confidence.

TWO HEMISPHERES, ONE HUMAN BEING

Our brains consist of two hemispheres with cross connections between them. This causes **the left hemisphere to control the right part of the body, and the right to control the left.** Damage to one of the hemispheres, e.g. due to a stroke, can lead to paralysis of the opposite side of the body.

> **Did you know ...?**
> In Western culture, we usually perceive time as flowing from the left (past) to the right (future). Research at the University of Geneva has shown that people who have a damaged right hemisphere have trouble thinking about the past (left side). In some tests, they attributed past events to the future.

Each of the brain hemispheres has tasks that it specializes in. Their execution is only possible when both hemispheres are functioning properly and there is unbroken communication between them. **Each of us simultaneously uses both hemispheres, thanks to the way in which the brain works properly** and we efficiently deal with our daily duties.

Example:
The left eye (right hemisphere) sees into afar, recognizes forms, colors, shapes, distribution in space and asymmetry. The right eye (left hemisphere) can see up close, see flat images and symmetry. Our ears have a different perception. It follows that only through synchronization, through the work of the entire body can integration in the process of perception and learning result.

Knowledge of the specializations of both hemispheres is important when choosing the correct brain exercises. If you want to improve your ability to think logically and you know that it is hidden in the left hemisphere of the brain, you can choose those exercises that will specifically encourage it's development.

The left hemisphere of the brain – the logical one

Thanks to this hemisphere, you can speak and understand what others say to you, perform mathematical calculations, recognize objects by touch and write. It is responsible for short-term memory and logical thinking, including:

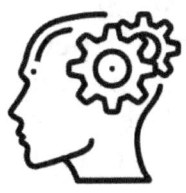

Analysis **Logic** **Sense of time**

 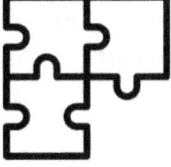 

The right hemisphere of the brain – the holistic one

Thanks to this hemisphere you can, amongst other skills, become an artist or create music. It is responsible for creative and abstract thinking. Without it we would not be able to read fluently, because it is there that the synthesis of letters and sentences takes place. In the right hemisphere, you will find:

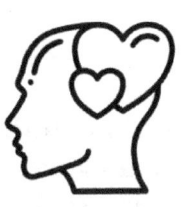

Intuition **Emotions** **Imagination**

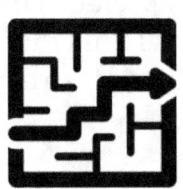 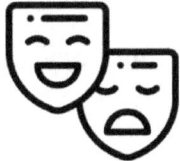 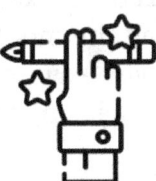

EXERCISE AND REMEMBER

„**Memory, the ability to gather information about things, events and experiences and to recall and use them at a later time,** is a process that occurs throughout the brain (there is more then one place for the storage of memories). This process involves creating new or reorganising the existing connections between cells.

Just as we can influence our physical condition and muscle mass through appropriate exercises, we can also influence our intellectual abilities. Thanks to mental exercises, we increase the number of connections between cells in the brain. **Memorization is a learned skill which can be trained and developed**, but which weakens if you do not practice it.

Studies have shown that in people regularly subjected to intellectual effort, the amount of enzymes responsible for breaking down proteins (considered one of the causes of Alzheimer's disease) increases."

- says Marcin Ratajczak, M.D.

Brain training activity does not have to be associated with physical exertion. Studies have shown that painting and other forms of art, such as learning to play an instrument, expressive or autobiographical writing, and learning a foreign language can also improve cognitive brain function. A 2014 study at Harvard University analyzed 31 exercises that focused on how these specific activities affected the mental abilities of older people. They all found that they improved several aspects of memory, such as rollback instructions and processing speed.

Neuroplasticity of the brain
It is the ability to learn and grow as the brain ages.
To utilize it you need to activate both hemispheres regularly.

NEW ACTIVITIES AS A REMEDY FOR BETTER MEMORY

New and difficult activity forces your brain to work on specific thought processes, such as problem solving and creative thinking. People aged 60 to 90 were selected for a psychological experiment in 2013. Some of them performed new and complex activities, such as digital photography or quilting. The second group dealt with things they had already known, such as reading and doing crosswords. It was proved that people from the first group, who devoted themselves to developing new skills for an average of 16 hours per week for three months, who achieved better results in work tests and long-term memory tests.

Practice is important.

„*It is the constant repetition of work on improvement, not the search for mastery, that might have the greatest impact*"

- dr Morris

Your activity should require a certain level of continuous practice, but striving for perfection is not your goal. The most important thing is the time you spend on engaging the brain in new challenges. You get more and more benefits with every minute you invest.

„*You cannot improve your memory if you don't work on it*"

- dr Morris

An exercise for you

Choose one new activity.
Enroll in class that interests you.
Plan your time for practice.
Make sure that you challenge your brain to develop. That is why choosing a new passion is so beneficial. It engages your brain to learn something new – you give yourself a chance to improve your memory and improve your quality of life!

Educational Kinesiology

A very important discovery by dr Paul Dennison, the creator of educational kinesiology, is **the identification of a close relationship between the condition of one's muscles and learning capability.** He has proven that a person experiencing stress has contracted, tense muscles, which blocks the flow of nerve stimuli, and thus hinders learning.

Kinesthetic sense (kinesthesia)	Feeling the position and movement of the limbs or parts of them relative to each other. Kinesthesia receptors inform the central nervous system about the nature and range of movements through the impulses they generate.
Kinesitherapy	Treatment with physical exercises, therapeutic gymnastics and massages.
Educational Kinesiology	A specialisation within the humanities concering the relationship between body movement and brain organization and functioning, with elements of psychology, pedagogy, neurophysiology and anatomy.

Note!
Our intelligence, learning skills and creativity do not depend on the weight and size of the brain or the number of nerve cells, as had been believed previously, but on **the number of connections between neurons.**

Coordinated movements offered by brain gymnastics affect the number and quality of connections between nerve cells. Thanks to this, the processes responsible for memory, concentration, creative thinking, writing, reading and correct pronunciation improve. It also eliminates excess stress and has a positive effect on body coordination.

Educational kinesiology is based mainly on movement, i.e. psychomotor exercises that improve the body, activate the nervous system, release stress-induced tension, and increase energy. The following 4 groups of exercises typical for brain gymnastics skill enhancement can be distinguished:

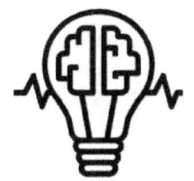
I. On crossing the midline

These exercises activate both hemispheres of the brain at the same time, stimulate the centers of speech and language in the brain, provide a „warm-up" for all skills that require crossing the brain's midline.

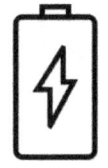
II. Energizing

These exercises activate the course of nerve processes between cells and groups of nerve cells in the brain and the body and have a direct impact on the physiological basis of receiving and remembering information.

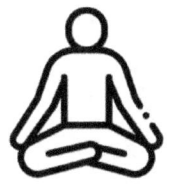
III. Relaxing

These exercises help to calm down, increase the positive attitude and gain motivation to act.

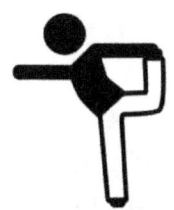
IV. Extending

These exercises limit the negative impact of the „tendon defense reflex" that arises when a new task is undertaken. They allow better communication between the posterior parts of the brain responsible for „survival" and the anterior (new cortex), where intellectual operations take place.

ACTIVATING EXERCISES
1. Alternating movements

Cross your arms and legs and integrate the hemispheres

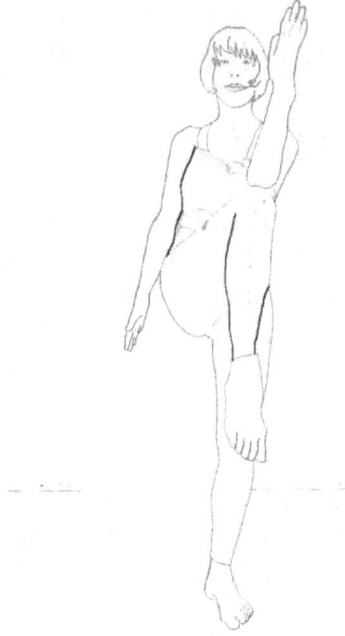

Description:

Raise the right knee and touch it with the left hand, then raise the left knee and touch it with the right hand, slightly twisting the whole body. This exercise resembles walking in place.

Purpose:

This exercise has a great impact on training the eye and removing its disorders. They activate both hemispheres to work simultaneously and constitute an excellent warm-up before further brain enhancing gymnastics.

2. Alternating movements – lying down

Alternating movements engages eyesight and hearing

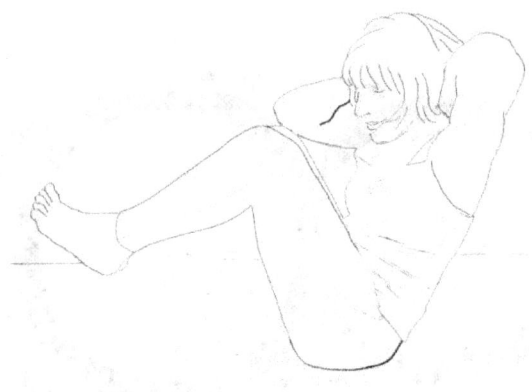

Description:

Do this exercise on a soft surface, in a horizontal position on the back. Knees and head are raised, arms folded behind the head to support it. Neck muscles relaxed, rhythmic breathing. Touch your elbow to the opposite knee, and then repeat the action with the other arm. Breathe rhythmically.

Purpose:

Integration of the right and left hemispheres and the right and left side of the body.

3. Lazy eights

Who practices the eights regularly can count on success!

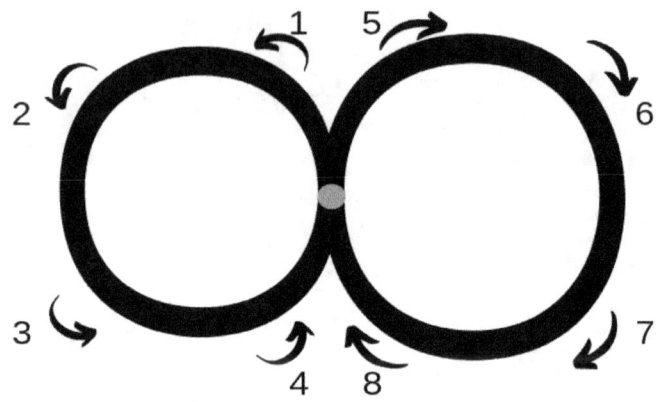

Description:

Set a point at eye level, opposite the nose. From there, start drawing a circle with the thumb upwards towards the left. When you return to the starting point, start drawing the second circle – upwards to the right. The eyes follow the movement of the hand. The drawing resembles an 8 lying on its side. Repeat this many times. Do it with alternating hands, then with both. Eights can be drawn in space, on the back of another person, on a wall, on paper, on sand...

Purpose:

Lazy eights improve vision and reading comprehension.

4. Alphabetical lazy eights

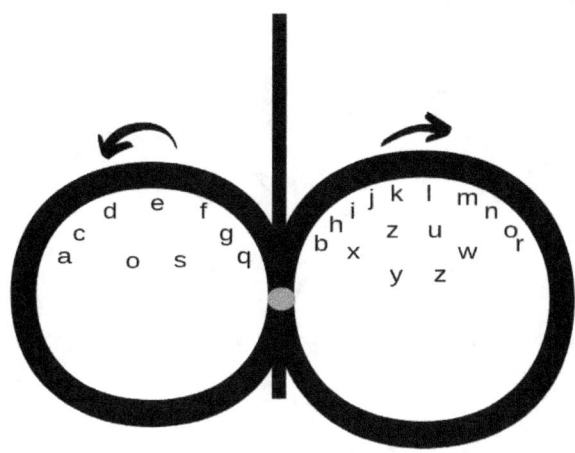

Description:

This is a modification of the „lazy eight". Draw a lazy eight, write in it lowercase letters of the alphabet in the left or right half, depending on the writing direction of the first segment of the letter, which is to consistent with the direction of drawing the eight. Draw a few lazy eights after each letter. You can do the exercise in the distance or on a flat surface.

Purpose:

This helps to learn the rules of spelling, affects creative writing, develops manual skills and precision of movements, allows to recognize and code symbols. Also improves eye-hand coordination.

5. Elephant

The elephant writes huge eights, sways his head and his trunk

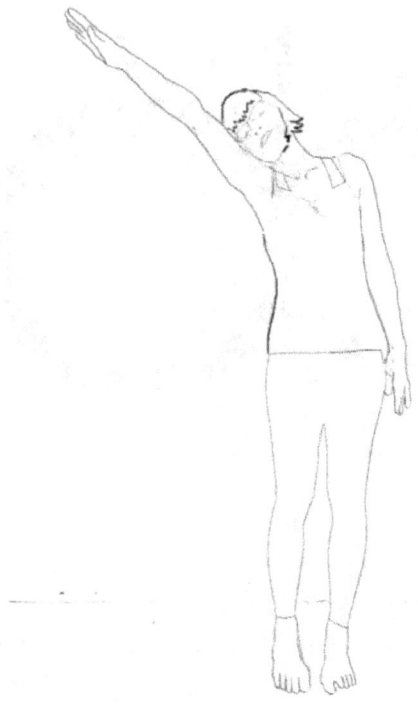

Description:

Stand with your legs slightly apart, the knees relaxed. With your arm stretched out and the back of your hand facing up, point to a focal point of the imaginary lazy eight in front of you. Press your ear to your shoulder and draw a lazy eight in space. The whole body works. Repeat the exercise three or four times with each arm.

Purpose:

To integrate hearing, vision and movement. This exercise coordinates the work of the brain's areas responsible for hearing in both hemispheres. It helps to develop long-term memory and corrects abnormal neck strains that arise when listening.

6. Diaphragmatic breathing

Description:

Take a deep breath. First, clean the lungs by breathing in through your lips pressed together (imagine you want to keep a feather in the air).
Then, you can breathe in even by the nose. Put your hands on the stomach, to rise on inhale, and go down on the exhale. Inhale and count to three, hold our breath for three seconds. Exhale and count to three, hold your breath for three seconds. Repeat the whole exercise once again.

Purpose:

This exercise teaches the proper breathing, so that the brain gets enough oxygen. This exercise relaxes the central nervous system and has a positive effect on the reading process.

7. Circling with the neck

Description:

Slowly move the head from shoulder to shoulder, allowing the chin to be as close to the chest as possible. Do it while exhaling. In the extreme lateral position of the head, breathe in and repeat the action.

Purpose:

Relaxation, reduction of neck muscle tension. Central nervous system relaxation. Activating the process of reading comprehension, expressing emotions, thinking, memory, calculating.

STRETCHING EXERCISES
1. Owl

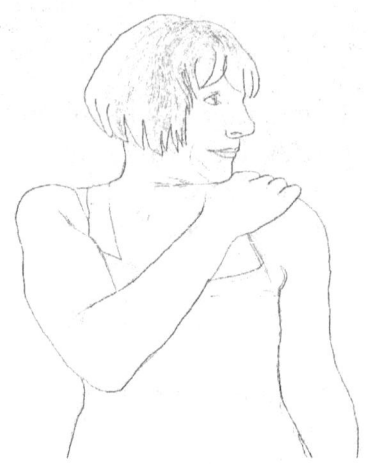

Description:

Firmly grasp the muscle on the left between the neck and shoulder with your right hand. Turn your head in this direction. Take a deep breath and exhale loudly while directing our head towards the opposite shoulder (you can articulate selected sounds or imitate the voice of an owl). When the head is over the right shoulder, take a deep breath again and exhale, returning to the starting point. Keep the head at the same height. After three to four cycles, repeat the exercise changing the arrangement of the hands.

Purpose:

This exercise reduces shoulder and neck muscle tension, which makes it easier for blood to reach the brain, which in turn allows for better concen-tration, focus attention faster and makes memory more efficient. Perception and memory, listening comprehension, speech and oral communication, mathematical calculations are all enhanced.

2. Active arm

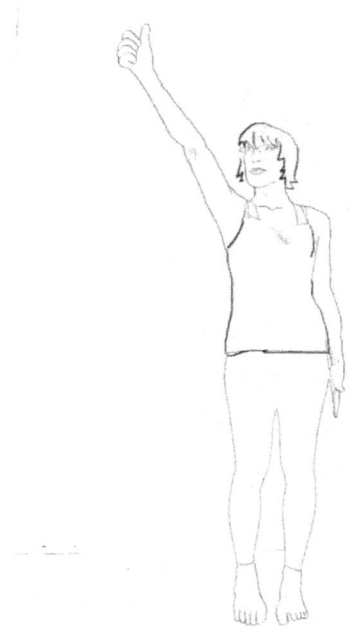

Description:

Raise your arm straight up. Grab it with the other hand from behind the head below the elbow and press in four directions as you exhale: towards the head, forward, backward, away from the ear. The raised hand resists the pressing hand. Repeat the exercise, changing hands.

Purpose:

This exercise allows you to stretch the upper muscles of the chest and arms. It is in this area that the use of these muscles in motor activity begins. Their shortening and tensions hamper such types of activity as writing or using tools. It affects the development of clear speech and language skills, relaxing the diaphragm, improves hand--eye coordination, improves calligraphy, spelling rules and creative writing.

3. Thinking points

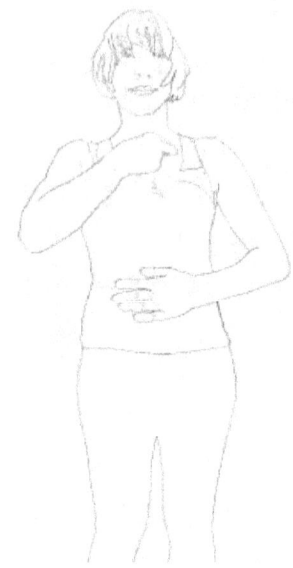

Description:

Put your left hand on the navel and use your right hand to massage the points just below the collarbone, on the left and the right side of the sternum. You can also tilt your head back and run your eyes along the line where the ceiling meets the wall.

Purpose:

Thinking points are the body's batteries.
They are favourable to the clarity of thinking, increase energy levels, and improve overall coordination and vision.

4. The COOC Position

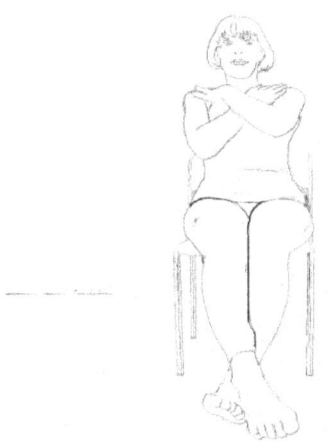

Description:

Part one: cross your legs at the ankles, weave the hands together and put them on the sternum, put your tongue on the palate, eyes closed. This position is considered to be the most effective one. You can do it while sitting, too.

Part two: feet are parallel to each other, fingertips are touching, tongue on the palate, eyes closed if you would like to relax. Return – open your eyes and breathe deeply.

Purpose:

This exercise provides increased concentration. Higher self-esteem. Correct pronunciation. The ability to listen carefully.

5. Relaxed bend

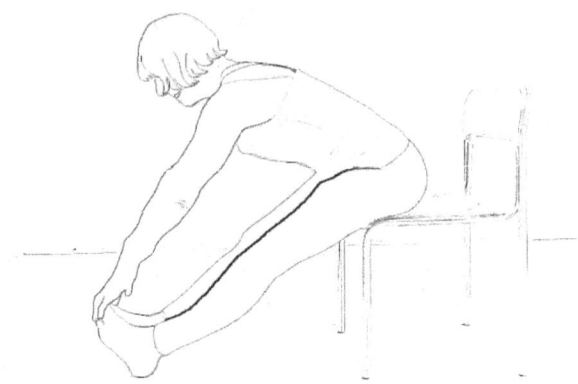

Description:

Sit down, with your legs stretched straight out and crossed at the ankles. Raise your hands, bend your torso forward. Inhale while doing the above, transferring body weight from one buttock to another several times. Hands and the body are on the same side. Exhale while straightning up. Repeat the exercise, changing the arrangement of the legs.

Purpose:

Feeling grounded and stable. Relaxation of the body. The exercise positively affects reading comprehension and mental calculation skills. A sense of balance and body coordination, increased confidence, increased visual concentration, deeper, energising breathing.

6. Heel pumping

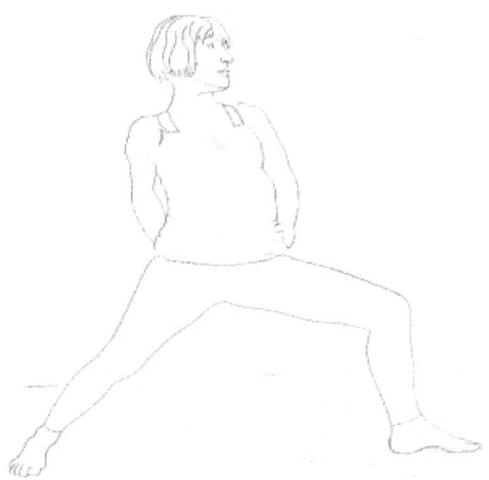

Description:

Stand behind a chair, hands firmly holding its back, step back with one leg. With an inhale, raise the foot of the extended leg to the toes, with an exhale lower it back so the heel touches the ground, bending the front leg in the knee. If you do not feel muscle tension during the exercise, increase the width of your step. Repeat the exercise several times slowly and smoothly, and then switch legs.

Purpose:

Integration of the anterior and posterior parts of the brain. Enhancing language skills.

7. A thinker's cap

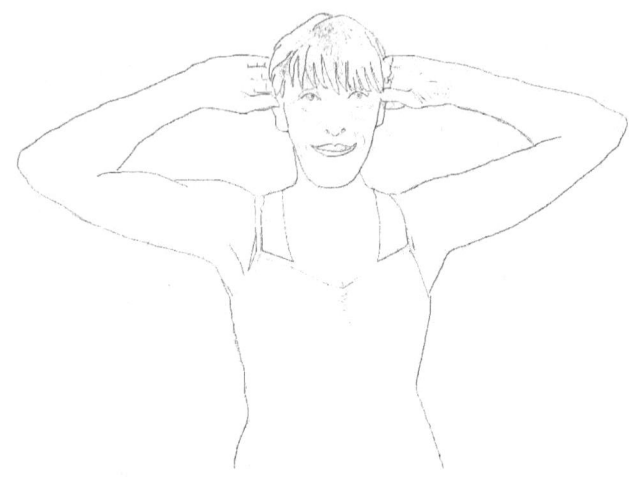

Description:

The exercise involves massaging the auricles, including stretching them out and turning them backwards, upwards and downwards. Repeat several times. The ear, which is shaped like an embryo, represents the entire body. By stimulating points on the auricle, we stimulate the whole body.

Purpose:

Recognizing sounds, careful listening, remembering sounds, hearing your own voice, increasing mental and physical fitness, stimulation of the inner ear, short-term working memory. The Thinker's Cap stimulates the hearing centers which disperse tones into individual sounds and combine them to obtain words or sounds with a specific meaning. At the same time, this exercise stimulates our imagination through music and rhythm.

8. Energetic yawning

Description:

Evoke yawning by massaging the mandibular joint with both hands at the same time. Lower the jaw slowly, pretending to yawn, making a deep, relaxing yawning sound.

Purpose:

This exercise shapes sensory perception, motor functions of the eyes and muscles responsible for sound and feeling, oxidation processes in the body, attention, visual perception, communication, the ability to select information, reading aloud, creative writing, public speaking.

9. Butterfly on the ceiling

Description:

Raise your head. With your nose, draw horizontal eights on the ceiling.

Purpose:

This exercise improves reading and writing skills.

CREATIVE EXERCISES
1. Word formation

Description:
Complete the words and add letters to the first syllables of the following words, so that new nouns, verbs or adjectives are formed.

Austr-	sho-	noteb-	boo-	bracel-	ca-	tig-	co-
turk-	less-	bak-	mat-	mant-	Bib-	Argenti-	com-
pavil-	car-	Wars-					

2. Read the following text aloud:
Peter Piper picked a peck of pickled peppers
A peck of pickled peppers Peter Piper picked
If Peter Piper picked a peck of pickled peppers
Where's the peck of pickled peppers Peter Piper picked?
Betty Botter bought some butter
But she said the butter's bitter
If I put it in my batter, it will make my batter bitter
But a bit of better butter will make my batter better
So 'twas better Betty Botter bought a bit of better butter

3. Memorising
Look at the words below for 4 minutes and try to remember them. Then cover the page and write down what you remember:

milk	f lour	bread	water	grains	gloves
scissors	scarf	Chicago	glass	Miami	heart

Create your own word lists to remember.

4. Drawing from memory
Look at this figure for ten seconds, then cover it with a piece of paper and draw it from memory:

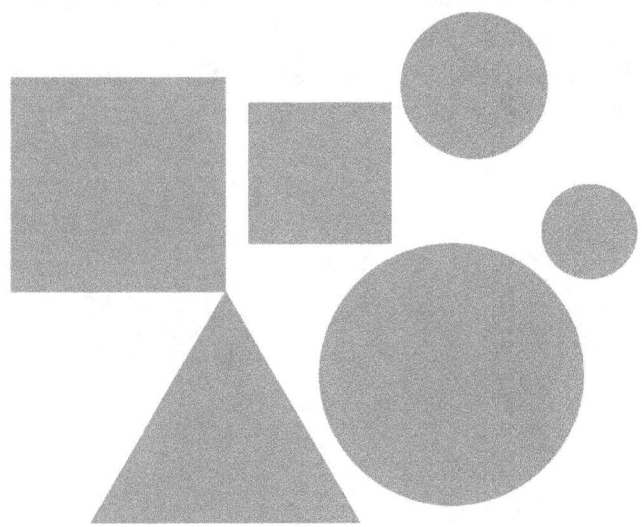

5. Hand exercise
Squeeze the fingertip of your right index finger firmly. Repeat with your middle, ring and little finger one by one. Repeat this exercise 20 times for each hand. Do this exercise twice a day. Try to change the pace.

6. Handwriting
Start writing by hand more, e.g. record your memories. One page every day. Prepare a shopping list or a daily to-do list. Write letters to friends. This exercise stimulates the brain and improves your nerve tissue's ability to create new connections.

7. Non-dominant hand exercises
Every day, do something with your non-dominant hand, e.g. brush your teeth, eat a meal, open the door. This will help to develop new connections between both hemispheres of your brain and strengthen the activity of the weaker hemisphere.

Your Guide to a Positive Life. Brain gymnastics for adults is the third collection in the series of original exercises. However, it is a complete Guide and you can work with it independent of the other volumes, thanks to which you will learn how to improve your brain's function to extend how long you can enjoy good memory and concentration, and acquire new skills.

The *Your Guide to a Positive Life* series is not a typical guide. You will not be bored with long pages of impractical advice or incomprehensible information. It is a notebook full of practical exercises that you will want to return to every day. Take the first step towards a more energetic life!

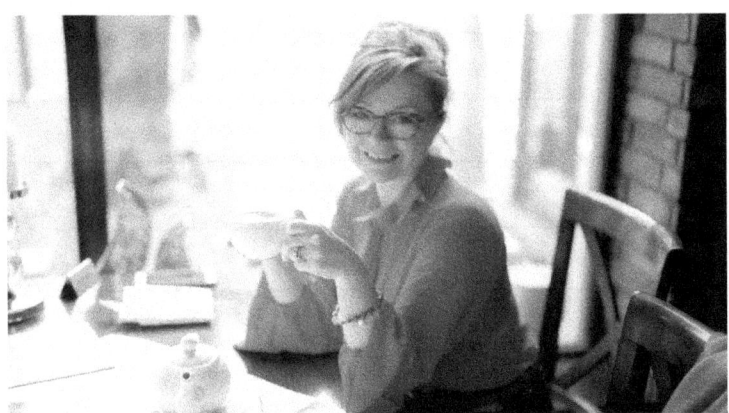

Foto: Beata Jastrzębska

Katarzyna Dorosz

A world-class expert working with the 50+ age group. She has worked for years to help change the lives of hundreds of people, infecting them with positive energy and motivating them to take the first step towards happiness and better health.

acti50.tv
katedorosz.com
Youtube - Acti50.tv
The Institute of Longevity - Instytut Długowieczności

www.ingramcontent.com/pod-product-compliance
Lightning Source LLC
Chambersburg PA
CBHW051413290426
44108CB00015B/2270